Review of the Revised Plan for Off-Site Treatment of Newport Chemical Agent Disposal Facility's Caustic VX Hydrolysate at DuPont Secure Environmental Treatment Facility in Deepwater, New Jersey

A Report to Congress

Prepared by:

Department of Health and Human Services

Centers for Disease Control and Prevention

July 2006 - *Corrected Version*

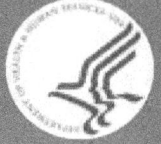

DEPARTMENT OF HEALTH AND HUMAN SERVICES

Centers for Disease Control and Prevention

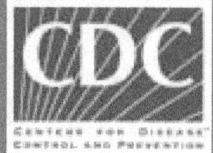

This page is intentionally blank

Table of Contents

This page is intentionally blank

SUMMARY

This report presents the findings of the follow-up review of the U.S. Army proposal for Caustic VX Hydrolysate (CVXH) waste transportation, treatment, and subsequent discharge of treated material into the Delaware River. The U.S. Army's plan for destroying their stockpile of bulk VX, a nerve agent developed for use in chemical warfare results in a treatment byproduct known as CVXH. The review was a joint effort by the Centers for Disease Control and Prevention (CDC) and the U.S. Environmental Protection Agency (EPA).

In a March 29, 2004, letter to CDC, the four U.S. Senators from New Jersey and Delaware, along with four members of the House of Representatives asked CDC to formally review the proposal for off-site treatment of CVXH to determine "if there is public health risk involved with the Army's proposal." This report, referred to as Phase I, identified several limitations of the available data that required resolution (1). They then asked both the U.S. Army and CDC to work together to address the remaining issues from the Phase I report and to review the proposed DuPont phosphonate removal process. The Army and DuPont conducted several studies and submitted the results to CDC and EPA for review. The findings of these reviews are as follows:

- In the Phase I review, CDC noted that the original treatment process proposed by DuPont had limited effectiveness in removing the phosphonate loading from the plant effluent. Because of the potential nutrient loading in the receiving waters, the Delaware River, DuPont proposed to augment their previously proposed treatment technology with additional processing to remove a major portion of the phosphonates from the plant effluent. DuPont conducted treatability studies on material produced in an Army laboratory before the start-up of the Newport Chemical Agent Disposal Facility (NECDF) and demonstrated that their process was effective in substantially reducing phosphonates in the effluent. A side benefit of the augmented process was the ability to effectively destroy any trace amounts of VX, if present, to below the detectible limits of the analytical equipment.
- In the Phase I review, CDC noted that clearance data (the ability to meet the VX and EA 2192 off-site shipment criteria as defined in Section 1) of this Report and treatability data for DuPont's treatment system was limited to the Newport process feed rate of 8% VX and for agent VX stabilized only with material known as diisopropylcarbodiimide (DIC). Clearance and treatability were

CDC's Approach

The review focused on three primary areas:

1) the information and test results required to address the findings and questions from the initial report to Congress,

2) a review of the feasibility of the phosphonate treatment proposal by DuPont and

3) future issues and concerns involving items such as the plans for process scale up, actual operations and managing process changes.

Conclusions:

If this project is approved by the regulatory officials, procedural requirements will need to be finalized to assure that all clearance and acceptance criteria specified by DuPont and the state of New Jersey are consistently met. Oversight and safeguard mechanisms, including management of change, sampling and communication between DuPont and NECDF will need continuing focus to ensure protection for public health and safety, and the environment throughout the life of the project.

subsequently demonstrated successfully for laboratory-generated feed stock for each feed/stabilizer variation identified in the Phase I report, as well as for a 16% laboratory generated material for all stabilizer variations

- In the Phase I review, EPA considered the data inadequate to assess the ecological toxicity associated with the DuPont plant discharge to the Delaware River. DuPont subsequently worked with EPA to develop a study protocol to produce the data needed by EPA to complete the assessment. The protocol was agreed upon by EPA in late June 2005, and the necessary tests were completed in August 2005 on the material produced (for the treatability tests mentioned above) from the laboratory-generated CVXH. EPA found that all of the previous ecological concerns have now been satisfactorily addressed by DuPont and/or the Army.

As the above concerns were being resolved, DuPont provided information on two other issues that were known to be of concern in the communities near their treatment facility. The first issue concerned the potential for Secure Environmental Treatment (SET) facility discharge into DuPont's Chambers Works plant effluent to affect area drinking water supplies as a result of discharging the treated CVXH. DuPont obtained and provided reports that examined local water basin characteristics, the location of water treatment plant intakes, and potential water quality impacts from area water discharge sources (2). DuPont provided data from models and tracer studies conducted in the 1980s and 1990s to describe flow and mixing characteristics of effluent from the DuPont Chambers Works plant under worst-case flow conditions. These studies supported the observation that the community water supplies in the area would not be adversely impacted by properly treated wastewater discharges from this plant.

DuPont, in cooperation with the Army, also evaluated the potential fate of VX and EA 2192 within and exiting the DuPont treatment process (3). While this material is regularly tested for VX below 20 parts per billion (ppb) and for EA 2192 below 1 part per million (ppm) at a non-detect per the method detection limit (MDL) criteria established by EPA, the community expressed concern that VX and EA 2192 could still be present. Tests conducted by the Army and DuPont demonstrated that the proposed phosphonate process is very effective in reducing the phosphonates and removing trace amounts of VX and EA 2192, to levels below established detection limits of the instruments used for the analysis.

During the gathering of data for this report, the Newport Chemical Agent Disposal Facility (NECDF) began full-scale destruction of VX at their site. This controlled start-up and associated developments provided CDC an opportunity to observe Newport's problem solving and management of process change capabilities, as well as their oversight and safeguard provisions.

Reviews conducted by CDC at DuPont, indicated that they have developed a waste characterization of the NECDF CVXH and identified characteristics that are critical to their treatment process. NECDF must consistently produce material to meet these criteria and maintain robust sampling and analytical techniques to confirm this to the satisfaction of the applicable regulations in the states involved. If key CVXH characteristics such as flammability, pH, or an increase in solids content change, CDC recommends that the regulators involved have the toxicology and transportation reevaluated to ensure public health and safety will not be compromised.

CDC and EPA developed the following new recommendations after reviewing the information provided by the Army and DuPont.

- NECDF should continue to collect performance data on representative sampling, and provide them to CDC for review, to maintain statistical confidence that representative hydrolysate samples are being collected consistently over time and from varying hydrolysate batches.
- Considering the potential need to re-characterize the CVXH, NECDF needs to develop an effective means to adequately sample the storage containers. CDC believes there is a need to determine what impact, if any, long-term storage will have on the material's characteristics and its conformance to the clearance criteria. In addition, DuPont will likely require new samples and analysis if storage of greater than one year occurs.

- EPA recommends that bioassessment studies be conducted in-stream by DuPont to establish baseline in-stream benthic macroinvertebrate and fish community structure in the vicinity, including downstream of the DuPont discharge, before CVXH processing begins.

Information Since Phase 1 Report

New data has been developed regarding:

1. Additional processing by DuPont for phosphonate removal from plant discharge.

2. Clearance and treatability of Newport CVXH produced by varied agent feed rates and for varying agent stabilizer combinations.

3. Toxicity testing to determine ecological impacts to the Deleware River, the receiving water for DuPont's plant effluent.

DuPont's modified process has been shown to be effective, on the laboratory scale, in removing phosphonates and eliminating trace amounts of VX and EA 2192 contaminants if needed. In the summer of 2005, DuPont completed testing done to meet EPA's data needs for assessing the potential ecological impact on the Delaware River. EPA has determined that all of its previous ecological concerns have been addressed by DuPont and/or the Army. If DuPont requests a modification of its current New Jersey Pollution Discharge Elimination System (NJPDES) permit for the acceptance of VX hydrolysate, EPA will act in its oversight role to ensure that the treated effluent meets the permit limitations set to protect the environment. Additionally, EPA will make every effort to provide relevant information and participate, as necessary, while DuPont proceeds with its ecological baseline project for the Delaware River.

In conclusion, CDC has found that the Army/DuPont proposal is sufficient to address critical issues in the areas of potential human toxicity, transportation, and treatment of CVXH. EPA has concluded that DuPont and/or the Army have addressed all of the previous ecological concerns. Consequently, CDC has no critical technical issues with the Army going forth with its plan to treat the NECDF-produced CVXH at an approved facility such as the DuPont SET.

INTRODUCTION

The U.S. Army has proposed a plan for destroying their stockpile of bulk VX, a nerve agent developed for use in chemical warfare. The proposed plan involves a multi-staged approach to the treatment, transportation, and disposal of the treatment byproducts.

The VX stockpile (1,269 tons in 1,690 containers) is currently stored and processed at the Newport Chemical Agent Disposal Facility (NECDF) in Newport, Indiana. The first stage of the plan is in process at this facility, where the VX is reacted with water and sodium hydroxide. The reaction results in a waste product referred to as caustic VX hydrolysate (CVXH).

The proposed second step is to transport the CVXH to another location, the DuPont Secure Environmental Treatment (SET) Chamber Works Facility in Deepwater, New Jersey, for secondary treatment. The DuPont facility will further treat the CVXH and then discharge the final waste product into the Delaware River. This proposal for CVXH transportation, treatment, and discharge into the Delaware River has raised concerns and questions about potential impacts on public health and the environment.

In a March 29, 2004 letter to the Centers for Disease Control and Prevention (CDC), the four U.S. Senators from New Jersey and Delaware, along with four members of the House of Representatives asked CDC to formally review the proposal for off-site treatment of CVXH to determine "if there is public health risk involved with the Army's proposal." In response to this request, CDC conducted the Phase I review. On April 6, 2005, CDC issued the Phase I report, *Review of the U.S. Army Proposal for Off-Site Treatment and Disposal of Caustic VX Hydrolysate from the Newport Chemical Agent Disposal Facility (1)*.

In the Phase I report, CDC stated that the proposal sufficiently addressed issues of human toxicity, treatment, and transportation of Newport CVXH; however, the U.S. Environmental Protection Agency (EPA) concluded that the information provided was inadequate to evaluate the ecologic risk associated with the discharge of the DuPont-treated CVXH into the Delaware River. The Phase I review also raised concerns that the level of phosphonates in the DuPont CVXH effluent being discharged into the Delaware River could encourage algae growth. In March 2005, DuPont provided CDC with new process information regarding a proposed method for reducing the levels of phosphonates in the effluent. This information was provided too late for consideration prior to issuance of the report on April

---

Introduction

On April 6, 2005, CDC issued the Phase I report, Review of the U.S. Army Proposal for Off-Site Treatment and Disposal of Caustic VX Hydrolysate from the Newport Chemical Agent Disposal Facility (1).

CDC did not recommend proceeding with the treatment and disposal at DuPont until EPA's noted deficiencies in the ecological risk assessment were addressed.

This report responds to those issues.

6, 2005. Members of Congress from New Jersey and Delaware requested that the Army and CDC work together to address the remaining issues from the Phase I report and review the proposed DuPont phosphonate removal process. They stressed the need for the completion of the independent review by CDC and public scrutiny of the findings.

> "We ask the Army and CDC to develop and advise us of the plan and schedule to complete the review [of the Army's proposal for off-site treatment of VX hydrolysate]…Let us be very clear, the process for treatment of the Newport hydrolysate cannot proceed until the review is completed, the findings made available for public scrutiny and all concerned understand precisely the risks involved and the potential impacts to the Delaware River."

This report responds to those requests.

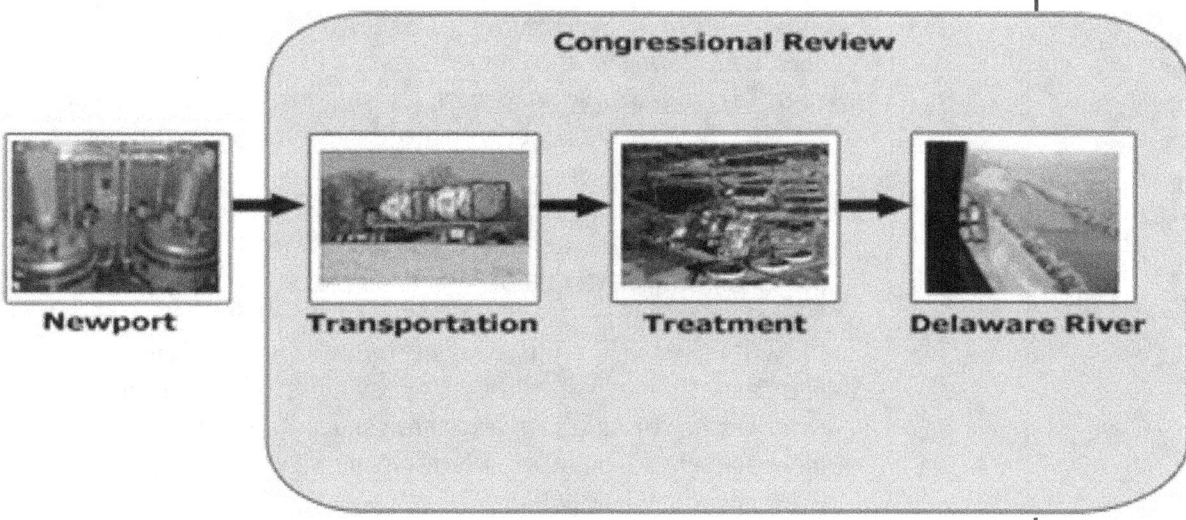

Shortly after receiving the latest request, CDC and the Army identified and selected key individuals in their respective organizations to assist with acquisition and analysis of the data required for this report. These individuals, along with EPA and DuPont representatives, engaged in a series of biweekly meetings to manage the identification, development, and submission of remaining data sets needed to complete CDC's review. Approximately half of the meetings were conducted face-to-face at locations alternating among the participants. The remaining meetings were conducted as conference calls. This method was effective in keeping data development on track and responsibilities clearly identified.

The review focused on three primary areas: a) the information and testing required to address the findings and questions from the initial report; b) a review of the feasibility of the phosphonate treatment proposal by DuPont; and c) plans and procedures in place to address future issues and concerns involving actions such as process scale-up, actual operations, and management of process changes.

EPA took the lead in reviewing the ecological toxicity data needed to examine the potential environmental impact of discharge of the DuPont-treated CVXH into the Delaware River. DuPont worked closely with EPA to identify appropriate test protocols needed to assess the acute and chronic toxicity potential associated with the New Jersey SET plant effluent.

Review

Congress requested the Army and CDC work together to address the remaining issues from the Phase I report and review the proposed DuPont phosphonate removal process. CDC worked with experts from Carmagen Engineering and the EPA to review and scrutinize Army and DuPont tests and data.

CDC and its contractor, Carmagen Engineering, took the lead in reviewing the treatability study data provided by DuPont. The resulting document, *Assessment of the Treatability of Caustic VX Hydrolysate at the DuPont Secure Environmental Treatment Facility (4)*, and DuPont's treatability study *(5)* are available on request. DuPont provided data to demonstrate the effectiveness of the modified process in removing phosphonates, and they provided data to evaluate their process effectiveness in treating a range of CVXH batches that varied by stabilizer mix and feed loading rate at the Newport plant. This was done to expand the confidence in the treatment process beyond that for the diisopropylcarbodiimide (DIC)-stabilized, 8% feed rate as examined in the Phase I report. All data developed for the Phase II report were available to all parties involved, regardless of which party took lead responsibility for its review. To ensure accurate and fair representation of data as reviewed, the generators of the data were provided the opportunity to comment on the assessment and bring factual inaccuracies to the attention of the authors of this report. CDC had the entire document peer reviewed prior to issuance.

CDC's charge was a) to address the findings and concerns from the Phase I review of the proposal to transport NECDF CVXH to DuPont's SET facility in Deepwater, New Jersey, for final treatment and subsequent discharge into the Delaware River and b) to review the proposed process for removal of phosphonates. In this Phase II report, the first section begins with a review of the recent developments with the NECDF process to neutralize the VX nerve agent, and then it addresses the requests from the members of Congress for review of the transportation, treatment, and discharge into the Delaware River. To properly analyze the proposed DuPont process, the review also focused on NECDF's ability to consistently produce hydrolysate that meets Army clearance and DuPont waste acceptance criteria.

Section 1. Review of VX Neutralization

NECDF Startup

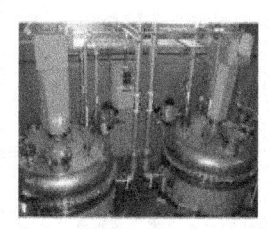

Newport

On May 5, 2005, NECDF began operations to chemically neutralize the nerve agent VX. This process was developed from laboratory bench-scale testing to determine if the technology was feasible for neutralizing the VX to levels below 20 parts per billion (ppb) and for minimizing formation of the key VX breakdown product, EA 2192, to levels below 1 part per million (ppm). The technology involves slowly adding the VX into a premixed volume or batch of a heated sodium hydroxide and water solution. The mixture is kept well mixed during this process to allow the VX to disperse and be effectively neutralized. The material produced during these laboratory-scale trials was the material used in the DuPont treatability studies and the subsequent aquatic toxicity studies.

The start-up of the pilot plant at NECDF yielded new process information along with expected and unexpected issues. The new process information yielded important insight that will assist in process-refinement in Newport. The plant, by the second week in June, had processed 24 separate batches of caustic VX hydrolysate. The data from samples of these batches (or "runs") demonstrated that the plant is capable of producing CVXH that meets the clearance criteria of less than 20 ppb of VX and less than 1 ppm of EA 2192. However, the sample results also provided new CVXH characterization data that required evaluation and comparison with the laboratory-produced CVXH used as the basis for the transportation and off-site treatment studies. For example, it was found that CVXH initially produced at NECDF's full-scale pilot plant exhibited the unexpected characteristic of flammability, which was not present in the laboratory bench-scale produced hydrolysate.

CVXH is primarily a caustic solution, but it does contain small amounts of combustible and flammable compounds such as diisopropylamine and ethanol. Although both diisopropylamine and ethanol represented less than one percent of the agent hydrolysate stream, testing indicated the material was flammable (flashpoint below 140 degrees Fahrenheit [°F]). As a result, the risk that flammable vapor might result from a large spill or leak could not be ruled out. This finding prompted the Army to commit to a means of eliminating this characteristic before allowing CVXH to be shipped off-site. On the basis of this testing, NECDF has three main criteria for shipment of CVXH:

- a non-detect for the method detection limit (MDL) (as defined by the EPA methods) of less than 20 ppb for VX,

- a non-detect for the MDL (as defined by the EPA methods) of less than 1 ppm for EA 2192, and

- a flashpoint (for determining flammability) of greater than 140 °F.

The potential differences in characteristics between the laboratory-scale testing and the production facility's product and in how the facility addressed these issues led to a review of how both NECDF and DuPont will respond to any future changes and ensure these changes do not adversely affect health and safety.

Concerns About Sampling System and Solids

The sampling system used at NECDF appears to be a sound design. However, restrictions in the piping, due to solids accumulation, affected the flow of material through the sampler numerous times during the initial startup of the facility. NECDF addressed this problem by modifying aspects of the design and operations six times within only a few months.

In their review, Carmagen identified three phases for CVXH: an organic phase (which contains the material diisopropylamine, ethanol, and other organic degradation products), a suspended solids phase, and an aqueous phase. To obtain a sample that accurately reflects or represents the contents of the reactor, the sample must be taken from a well-mixed flow of material that is not allowed to separate.

In addition to the problem of sampling restrictions, Carmagen was concerned that the solids could contain high concentrations of VX, thereby impacting the analysis and increasing public risk. At the recommendation of CDC, the Army had some of the solid material tested at an outside laboratory. The analysis indicated the solids contained 1 ppm or less of VX, which was similar to the values previously reported for the organic layer of the CVXH. Based on current waste characterization by DuPont, the solids content is well below 0.02 percent, and the contribution of VX in the solids to the overall sample would be negligible. CDC determined that the public health impact is negligible at those concentrations.

From the reactor, CVXH is then pumped to a hydrolysate holding tank near the reactor in the Toxic Cubicle, where it is held until the sample results are available. After assurance that the specifications have been met, the CVXH is pumped to a large tank outside the Toxic Cubicle, where it is mixed with other batches to produce enough material to fill an isotainer or other shipping container. The reactor sample provides the final determination that the reaction is complete, that is, a non-detect for the MDL (as defined by EPA methods) below 20 ppb for VX, a non-detect for the MDL (as defined by EPA methods) below 1 ppm for EA 2192, and a flashpoint (for determining flammability) above 140 °F. This determination of the reaction's "completeness" in meeting the shipping specifications for VX, EA 2192, and the flashpoint is referred to as "cleared" or "clearance."

In addition to indicating whether the batch has cleared, this sample is used to determine the waste characteristics identified by DuPont for shipment and is used as the shipping sample. The analysis of the shipping sample (waste characterization) provides the information to the treatment, storage, and disposal facility (DuPont SET) to set the parameters for its treatment of the CVXH.

As stated previously, restrictions or plugging of the system can result in samples that are not representative of the contents of the reactor used to neutralize the VX. In other process designs, such an issue would not be as significant, because the samples could be taken in other locations downstream to verify the material characteristics of the reactant product. However, for this design, the reactors are the most efficiently agitated vessels in the NECDF system and, therefore, the only locations where well-mixed, representative samples can be obtained. The sampling system for the reactors is of critical importance because of NECDF's design and operational plan.

During the start-up of the facility, several incidents occurred during which tanks were contaminated when manual tank valves were incorrectly operated or automatic valves failed to function correctly. These incidents were detected, the material isolated, and corrective actions planned to prevent reoccurrence. As stated previously, no means currently exist for NECDF to resample these vessels (storage tanks) to determine the impact of the contamination. NECDF plans to return any such material to the reactors for reprocessing as needed.

On the basis of good technical and operating practice, NECDF should have an additional method to allow representative sampling from storage tanks and shipping containers if there is concern that the sampler had not functioned correctly or to verify the CVXH characteristics have not changed due to long-term storage or possible contamination. Currently, if the material needs to be rechecked or verified, the only way to obtain a sample is to return the material to the reactor. Such action is a long and complex process that reduces the facility's available production capacity. Although NECDF has increased the operational reliability of the sampler, no downstream backup or verification is in place. CDC recommends that NECDF develop a plan to address this deficiency in the design and operation of the system.

Summary of Carmagen's Report on NECDF Process Status

NECDF was designed to be operated initially as a pilot-plant facility because the process had been demonstrated only at a laboratory/bench scale. During plant operations, therefore, it is not unexpected that significant changes may be required before the NECDF is considered to be "production-ready." After reviewing the process status, CDC and its contractor made the following conclusions.

- The NECDF facility is capable of processing VX to produce a hydrolysate that meets all requirements for shipment to the DuPont SET facility.

- NECDF uses the reactor sampling system and laboratory analytical methods to verify that CVXH clearance criteria have been met. The efficacy of the reactor sampling system is critical to ensure that CVXH meets these criteria. Because downstream storage tanks and containers cannot be effectively mixed, a representative sample cannot be readily obtained for confirmatory analysis after the CVXH is discharged from the reactor to these locations.

Summary of Carmagen's Report on NECDF Analytical Methods

The primary purpose of this review and evaluation was to define the adequacy of the currently proposed methods for the sampling and analysis of VX and EA 2192 in the CVXH to meet NECDF programmatic clearance requirements. The scope of this review covered the sampling, laboratory analyses, and related quality assurance/quality control (QA/QC) of dicyclohexyldicarbodiimide (DCC), DIC, and DIC/DCC-stabilized VX hydrolysate at the 16% VX loading levels.

In the Phase I report, issues were raised with the Army's use of MDLs for clearance, but it was stated: "While CDC believes that utilizing the MDL approach would not result in public health concerns, the Army needs to address potential public misperceptions regarding the detection or non-detection of VX in CVXH." Furthermore, CDC believed that the Army's clearance criteria of "non-detect with an MDL less than an established concentration level" combines two related, but different, analytical chemistry concepts. The first concept is that of instrument or analytical detection, which is a qualitative-based criterion, and the second concept is that MDL is a statistically calculated, quantitative criterion.

In the Phase II review by Carmagen, concerns about the MDL were again noted, specifically in relation to the use of a global MDL and, given the low instrument detection limits, the spike levels used. One noted outcome was a calculated limit of quantification (LOQ) that was above the clearance criteria of 20 ppb, which is statistically undesirable. The LOQ is defined as the lowest level or concentration for which numerical results may be obtained with a specified degree of confidence. These issues were determined not to impact the overall capability of the laboratory to meet the clearance specifications, or the risk to public health. However, the Army's use of such terms can still lead to misperceptions and therefore require additional clarification. Additional information about current developments regarding the MDL, LOQ, and other analytical concepts is available on EPA's Web site (http://www.epa.gov/ost/methods/det/).

These reviews (4) resulted in the following findings and recommendations:

Findings

- The design of the reactor, current mixing systems, sampling system, and planned mass flow monitoring systems, working in conjunction with current sampling protocols and quality-control measures, are capable of providing representative hydrolysate samples to the NECDF laboratory for clearance analyses. Also, current procedures and protocols in place for sub-sampling the plant sample in the laboratory can provide adequate final analytical samples for clearance analyses. NECDF needs to generate adequate QA/QC analytical data to confirm over time and with varying hydrolysate batches the performance of these two sampling events.

- The current methods for analyzing VX and EA 2192 in 16% VX loaded, DIC, DCC, and DIC/DCC stabilized CVXH have demonstrated the capability to ensure that the hydrolysate meets Army clearance specifications.

- The NECDF laboratory's QA/QC plans and procedures for monitoring, defining, and controlling the analyses of the CVXH for VX, EA 2192, and other characterization analytes are well designed and documented.

Moving Forward

Statistical confidence in hydrolysate sampling and analysis needs to be assured throughout the life of this project.

NECDF should have a clear, planned means to provide representative sampling of on-site, stored hydrolosate as the need arises.

Recommendations

- NECDF should continue to collect performance data on representative sampling, and provide them to CDC for review, to maintain statistical confidence that representative hydrolysate samples are being collected consistently over time and from varying hydrolysate batches.

- Considering the potential need to re-characterize the CVXH, NECDF needs to develop an effective means to adequately sample the storage containers. CDC believes there is a need to determine what impact, if any, long-term storage will have on the material's characteristics and its conformance to the clearance criteria. In addition, DuPont will likely require new samples and analysis if storage of greater than one year occurs.

Section 2. Review of Transportation

Toxicology and Transportation Review

On the basis of testing conducted during this review and the subsequent identification and resolution of the flammability issue, CDC believes that the toxicology and transportation analyses contained in the Phase I report are still valid for material that meets the criteria proposed by DuPont for CVXH. Additional data have been provided to supplement the treatability concerns identified during the Phase I review. That is, chemical processing technology being used by NECDF has been duplicated on a laboratory scale and demonstrated that it can treat variations in agent VX feed rates and stabilizer mix and produce material that meets the current criteria for shipment to the DuPont facility. Furthermore, treatability for these laboratory-generated variations has also been confirmed through a laboratory-scale simulation of the DuPont SET process (5).

Since issuance of the Phase I report, CDC became aware of community questions or concerns regarding the toxicity impacts of any residual stabilizers (DIC or DCC) or other residual decomposition products in the CVXH. CDC was unable to locate substantial studies or data to address these questions. CDC recognizes that there will always be some variation in the minor components of CVXH between agent lots and individual process batches.

On the basis of data supplied by the Army and DuPont, CDC concludes that the Army's clearance criteria, coupled with DuPont's acceptance criteria, provide an adequate foundation to characterize and manage the risks associated with shipping CVXH. The major risk with CVXH, even at the 16% loading, remains corrosivity. Protective measures planned for responses to a spill event involving strong corrosives are the primary safeguards for personnel exposure and protection. These measures should also be adequate to protect against contact with material that could potentially contain small amounts of toxic byproducts.

Potential changes in the material characteristics as defined in Section 3, Review of Treatment at DuPont, may be sufficient to warrant an update of the toxicology and transportation assessments. These assessments were based on DuPont's waste characterization profile and their requirement that shipments meet this profile.

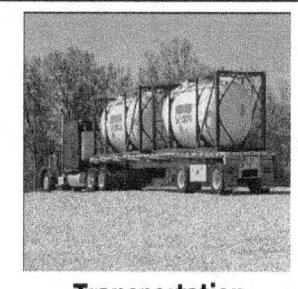

Transportation

Over-the-Road Transport

NECDF identifies 3 main criteria for shipment of CVXH:

1. Non-detect for the MDL ≤ 20 ppb VX
2. Non-detect for the MDL ≤ 1 ppm EA 2192
3. Flashpoint > 140 degrees

Note that DuPont's waste characterization profile does not allow for flammable material and that flammability was not considered for these assessments. The Army and NECDF made a commitment to not ship flammable material offsite, even though no regulatory requirement prohibits such shipment. CDC based its evaluation on that commitment and on the progress demonstrated in resolving the issue. If key CVXH characteristics such as flammability, pH, or an increase in solids content change, CDC recommends that the regulators involved have the toxicology and transportation reevaluated to ensure public health and safety are not compromised.

Section 3. Review of Treatment at DuPont

Summary of Carmagen's Report on CVXH Treatment at DuPont

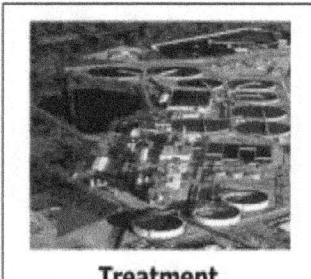

Treatment

After transportation to the DuPont SET facility, CVXH is treated by a series of physicochemical and biologic processes to adjust the pH and remove the organic by-products. The objective of the review and evaluation of the phosphonate removal treatability study and basic data addendum was to determine if the DuPont SET facility could successfully treat 16% VX loaded CVXH while addressing the community's concerns about the potential impact of phosphonates (ethyl methylphosphonic acid [EMPA] and methylphosphonic acid [MPA]) in the effluent released into the Delaware River.

Findings

- The DuPont combined pretreatment studies demonstrate that 16% VX loaded CVXH DIC, DCC, and DIC/DCC stabilized hydrolysate can be effectively treated to remove phosphonates (EMPA and MPA) before biotreatment. The results of the testing are shown in Figure 1 (5).

Figure 1. Removal Efficiency of the DuPont Revised Process

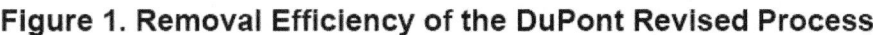
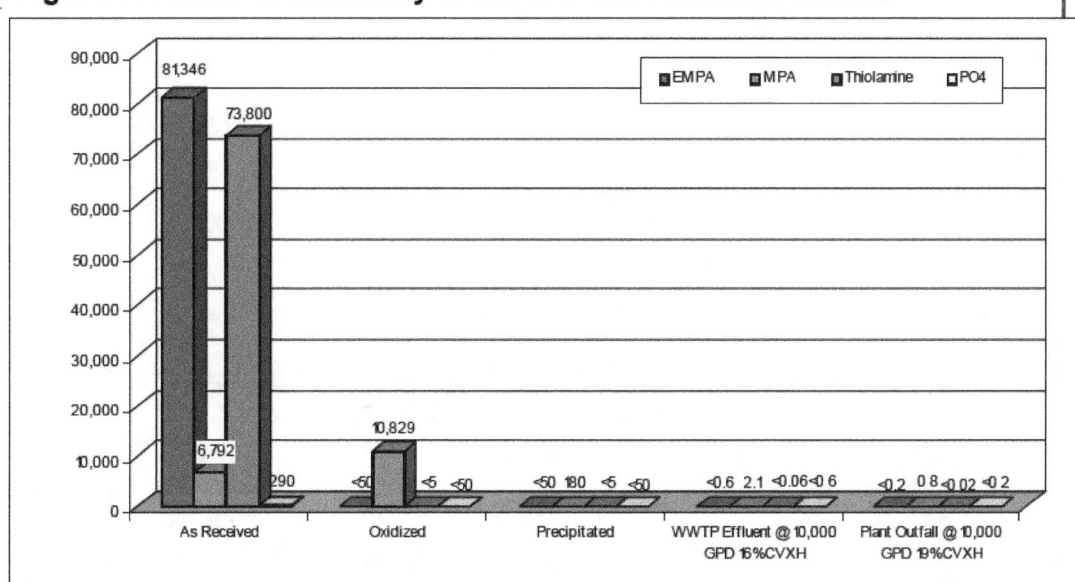

Key: mg/L = micrograms per liter; EMPA = ethyl methylphosphonic acid; MPA = methylphosphonic acid; PO4 = phosphate; WWTP = wastewater treatment plant; GPD = gallons per day; NCH = Newport (Indiana) caustic hydrolysate.

Adapted from E.I. DuPont & Company. Treatability study summary for phosphonate removal technology on 16% Newport (IN) caustic hydrolysate. Wilmington, Delaware: E.I. DuPont & Company; Aug 2005.

- The biotreatability study demonstrates that the DuPont SET facility can accept 16% VX loaded CVXH DIC, DCC, and DIC/DCC combined pretreated hydrolysate without process upsets or a measurable drop in treatment performance.

- The DuPont peroxide/persulfate oxidation treatment process study has demonstrated the ability of the process to destroy VX and EA 2192 to levels below the limits of analysis in 16% VX loaded CVXH DIC stabilized hydrolysate.

- DuPont has the experience and process-safety management requirement procedures in place to scale-up and implement the persulfate oxidative combined pretreatment process demonstrated in the laboratory at their SET facility.

Treatment

DuPont's tests have shown them to be capable of successfully treating the currently anticipated CVXH variations.

DuPont's waste acceptance profile criteria ensures that CVXH remains conformant and compatible with their treatment process.

Section 4. EPA Review

Ecological Impacts to the Delaware River

In April 2004, Region 2 of the United States Environmental Protection Agency (EPA) was asked by the Centers for Disease Control and Prevention (CDC) to assist with the review of the Army's proposal to treat VX hydrolysate at DuPont's Chambers Works SET wastewater treatment plant in southern New Jersey and discharge the treated effluent to the Delaware River. Previous to this CDC request, the Army's proposal and draft Environmental Assessment Statement (EAS) and Finding of No Significant Impact (FONSI) were reviewed by Delaware's Department of Natural Resources and Environmental Control (DNREC), the Delaware River Basin Commission (DRBC), and the New Jersey Department of Environmental Protection (NJDEP). Their concerns about the proposal included treatment capacity of the SET and potential effects of phosphorus and residual VX on the estuary.

EPA's role in the review process focused only on potential ecological effects of the DuPont proposal in the Delaware River. Human health risks as well as the potential risks from the destruction process and transportation were assessed by the CDC and others. Moreover, EPA was not asked to evaluate other possible alternatives for VX destruction and disposal. Finally, EPA's evaluation of project information was premised on assurances by the Army Chemical Materials Agency (CMA) that the hydrolysate being shipped to DuPont will not contain detectable levels of VX and EA 2192 and will not be flammable. DuPont has stated that it will not accept any hydrolysate that does not meet these parameters.

EPA's Review and Findings

In its October 2004 comments on the DuPont Screening Level Ecological Risk Assessment (SLERA), EPA stated that the report "… does not contain adequate information to conclude that there is no unacceptable risk from the discharge of treated VX hydrolysate to the Delaware River." EPA's position was that "… DuPont has not demonstrated that the disposal of material as presented in the ecological risk assessment is acceptable."

Over the course of more than a year, DuPont and the Army CMA have performed studies and prepared reports to address EPA's concerns. EPA's concerns were divided into five major topics dealing with conservatism,

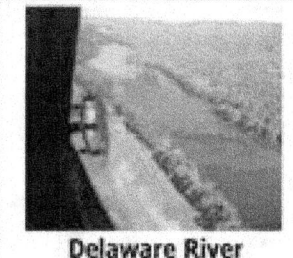
Delaware River

Background

In Phase 1 of this review, EPA did not have adequate data to assess ecological impacts to the Deleware River from the discharge of treated CVXH. This report reviews the new data developed to meet EPA's needs.

toxicity test issues, the potential presence of VX and other toxic breakdown products in the hydrolysate, the addition of phosphorus to the Delaware River, and National Pollutant Discharge Elimination System (NPDES) permit issues. The full text of EPA's comments can be found in the Phase I CDC report dated April 2005. A summary of EPA's five major ecological concerns, the efforts by project participants to address those concerns, and the Agency's subsequent findings are listed below.

Item 1 from the Phase 1 Report - The SLERA lacks conservatism

EPA Concern

EPA's concerns included the need to evaluate all detected constituents at their maximum concentration in the risk calculations, account for unidentified constituents, eliminate the use of dilution factors in estimating constituent concentrations, and recalculate the Hazard Indices for constituents having similar ecological effect endpoints and/or toxic mechanisms. EPA reviewed the DuPont SLERA consistent with the approach it would use for screening level ecological risk assessments for a Superfund hazardous waste site or Resource Conservation Recovery Act (RCRA) corrective action facility. Although it was called a SLERA, DuPont's original report did not contain many of the conservative assumptions that EPA expects to be used in hazardous waste program-specific risk assessments meant to characterize potential ecological risks.

Response

Subsequent to the preparation of the SLERA, DuPont performed acute aquatic toxicity tests that assessed whether the proposed treatment technologies could produce an effluent that would meet the existing NPDES permit limit for whole effluent toxicity (WET) of an LC50 greater than the 50% effluent. DuPont ran acute and chronic toxicity tests on 8% and 16% hydrolysate mixtures that appropriately considered EPA's concerns. WET testing assesses the combined effects of all the constituents found in the wastewater treatment plant effluent at their maximum concentrations including chemicals that cannot be identified through chemical analysis. The standardized procedures of WET tests allow for the determination of adverse biological effects using the species representing three different trophic levels. Toxicity tests measure the aggregate effects of all constituents in a wastewater, including the interactions of all chemicals in the complex mixture, including those known or not detectible using routine chemical analysis.

Finding

- EPA has reviewed the laboratory studies and reports prepared by DuPont and the Army since October 2004 and determined that its ecological concerns about the Delaware River and estuary have been addressed. The whole effluent toxicity testing done by DuPont provides a level of information and certainty far beyond what would be expected in a SLERA, so there is no need to revise that SLERA itself. The issue concerning the use of dilution factors in the estimation of in stream concentrations of constituents is no longer applicable because the toxicity tests measure adverse organism effects using the concentrations of the chemicals actually present in the effluent regardless of mixing with water from the Delaware River.

Item 2 from the Phase I Report - Toxicity Test Issues

EPA Concern

Concerns with the toxicity tests included limited effluent concentrations used in testing, the need to perform the tests on three species, the need to perform chronic testing on the final CVXH effluent using three species, and the use of quality control procedures as outlined in the EPA acute and chronic testing manuals (EPA 2002, 2002a & 2002b) in order for the data to be acceptable.

Response

DuPont performed additional toxicity tests which included retesting the acute exposures and conducting chronic toxicity tests with three species representing three trophic levels:

- *Pimepheles promelas*, fathead minnow
- *Ceriodaphnia dubia*, water flea
- *Pseudokirchneriella subcapitata* (formerly *Selenastrum capricornutum*), unicellular green algae

All quality control procedures as outlined in EPA's *Short-Term Methods for Estimating the Chronic Toxicity of Effluents and Receiving Waters to Freshwater Organisms, 4th edition* (821-R-02-013, October 2002) were followed.

The chronic testing was conducted in three series:

- Series 1— Effluent from the pretreatment process at 8% CVXH and 16% CVXH, both concentrations were tested using the three different stabilizers (DIC, DCC, and DIC/DCC).

- Series 2— Effluent resulting from the patented Powdered Activated Carbon Treatment System (PACT®) biotreatment with 8% CVXH (DIC only) and 16% CVXH (DIC, DCC, and DIC/DCC) at two different loading rates of 5,000 and 10,000 GPD.

- Series 3— Artificial effluent prepared to mimic the major salt ions (calcium, magnesium, sodium, chloride, sulfate, and bicarbonate) found in the PACT® biotreatment effluent.

The DuPont SET currently does not have chronic testing as part of its NPDES permit. In order for the tests results to be acceptable, the No Observable Effective Concentration (NOEC) must be greater than the in-stream waste concentration (IWC) determined by the Delaware River Basin Commission (DRBC) as 0.4%. All chronic test results were above this limit.

The most sensitive species was *C. dubia* when exposed to 16% CVXH pretreatment effluent with DCC stabilizer (series 1), and 16% NCH PACT® treated effluent with DIC and 10,000 GPD (series 2). The NOEC for both tests was 3.1% which is greater than the IWC of 0.4%. This effect was also mimicked in the artificial effluent (series 3) for the same conditions.

Findings

- These tests along with tests from the Treatability Study are an acceptable demonstration that the proposed pretreatment and PACT biotreatment of CVXH when processed alone should not cause any adverse conditions upon discharge into the Delaware River.

- DuPont plans on alternating the processing of CVXH through the PACT® system with other wastes such as Aberdeen caustic hydrolysate (ACH). These chronic tests conducted to date do not take into consideration any chemical constituents which may remain in the PACT®. The ability to conduct such tests will not present itself until the actual alternate processing of the CVXH and ACH begins.

Recommendation

- Accordingly, EPA recommends that bioassessment studies be conducted in-stream to establish baseline in-stream benthic macroinvertebrate and fish community structure in the vicinity, including downstream of the DuPont discharge, before CVXH processing begins. A team, with members from EPA, New Jersey Department of Environmental Protection (NJDEP), Delaware River Basin Commission (DRBC), Delaware Department of Natural Resources and Environmental Control (DNREC), and DuPont should be established to design the ambient study and monitor the final processing of CVXH. In fact, recent correspondence that EPA has received from DuPont indicates that the company has already taken initial steps to assemble ecological baseline data from various participants in their Delaware River Estuary project.

Item 3 from the Phase I Report -VX nerve agent and other toxic breakdown products could be present in the hydrolysate.

EPA Concern

EPA expressed concern that VX nerve agent, EA 2192, and other toxic breakdown products might be present in the treated hydrolysate and that there is no information demonstrating that the SET is capable of treating VX nerve agent or EA2192.

Response

An Army study and subsequent report, *Effect of the DuPont Persulfate Treatment Process on Trace Quantities of VX and EA2192 in Hydrolysate* (August 2005) (*3*), addresses EPA's concerns about the potential for the presence of VX and other toxic breakdown compounds in the hydrolysate. Known amounts of VX and EA 2192, an order of magnitude higher than the MDLs and hydrolysate clearance criteria, were added to the hydrolysate and treated under the conditions of the DuPont process. The results of the study demonstrated that the persulfate oxidative treatment proposed by DuPont to destroy thiolamine and EMPA would also destroy any trace amounts of VX and EA 2192 in the hydrolysate to levels below the limits of analysis.

The report concluded that the DuPont proposed peroxide/persulfate oxidation process completely destroys VX and EA 2192 in 16% hydrolysate. According to DuPont, levels of VX and EA 2192 in the hydrolysate transported and treated at the Chambers Works facility will not be detectable. Moreover, DuPont has stated that it would not accept waste containing detectable levels of VX and EA 2192.

DuPont's October 2005 report, *The Fate of VX, EMPA, MPA, and Other Constituents in Newport Caustic Hydrolysate* describes the path the constituents will take from the Newport, Indiana facility through the SET plant at the Chambers Works site. DuPont estimates that the neutralization process in Newport will decrease VX in the hydrolysate from an initial concentration of 80,000 parts per billion (ppb) to non-detect (<20ppb) within 150 minutes at a temperature of 90°C. Using first order reaction equations, the resulting concentration of VX is estimated to be $6.6 \times 10\text{-}32$ ppb, which is significantly less than the 20 ppb detection limit. Wastewater containing this extremely low level of VX would be further treated at the DuPont SET facility using oxidative persulfate oxidative pretreatment, precipitation, and biological treatment. As described above, any trace amounts of VX present in the hydrolysate will be further destroyed by the proposed persulfate oxidative pretreatment.

Finding

- EPA believes that with the addition of DuPont's proposed persulfate oxidative treatment process to the Chambers Works facility's treatment regime, the SET will be capable of reducing any levels of VX or EA2192 that could potentially be present.

Item 4 From the Phase I Report - The addition of phosphorus to the Delaware River could be detrimental.

EPA Concern

EPA found the original report unclear concerning the effect of the addition of MPA and other phosphorus-containing compounds from the discharge of the treated caustic VX hydrolysate effluent into the Delaware River. The agency's principal concern was that the discharge of these compounds could increase the amounts of dissolved inorganic phosphorus in the estuary to such a point that the system would create unwanted algal blooms.

Response

In March 2005, DuPont submitted the *Treatability Study for Phosphonate Removal Technology* to EPA for consideration. This report demonstrated that their new treatment process removes approximately 99% of the phosphonate compounds during the treatment of the caustic VX hydrolysate. This report was reviewed by both EPA regional staff and the Office of

Research and Development (ORD). Although our review revealed some minor errors, we agreed with the conclusions.

The DuPont report, *Treatability Study Summary for Phosphonate Removal Technology on 16% Newport (IN) Caustic Hydrolysate* was submitted to the EPA in August 2005.

The object of the report was to determine if the SET facility could successfully treat 16% caustic VX hydrolysate containing the three different stabilizers. The report concluded that the combined pre-treatment involving persulfate oxidation and ferric chloride precipitation removes greater than 97% of the phosphonates (EMPA and MPA) from the waste-stream before it enters the wastewater treatment plant.

Finding

- EPA concerns regarding the addition of phosphorus-containing compounds to the Delaware River are adequately addressed by the protocols and procedures used in the proposed phosphonate-removal treatment that DuPont will add to the ultimate treatment of VX hydrolysate before it enters the river.

Item 5 from the Phase I Report - NPDES Permit Issues.

EPA Concern

DuPont's Chambers Works facility discharges wastewater into the Delaware River under the terms, conditions, and provisions of a NPDES permit that is administered by NJDEP. The NJDEP is the delegated permitting authority for discharges in the State of New Jersey. EPA's role in the NPDES program involves oversight of New Jersey State's NPDES permitting program. At the time of EPA's Phase I comments, the NPDES permit for the Chambers Works facility (NJ0005100) had expired on January 31, 2004 and did not include a limit or a requirement to monitor and report on MPA, thiolamine,

and EA2192. EPA was concerned that the Army's proposal would be considered a major alteration as defined in 40 CFR 122.62 (a) (1) since the addition of this wastestream will result in changes in the permittee's practices that are different in the DuPont NPDES renewal application.

Response

NJDEP issued a renewal permit (NJ0005100) for the DuPont Chambers Works facility on August 10, 2005; the effective date is October 10, 2005 with an expiration date of September 30, 2010. Effluent limitations were included in the permit to address the facility's discharge of process wastewater, stormwater, cooling water, groundwater remediation wastewater, leachate, and wastewater delivered from offsite facilities.

The permit specifically prohibits the acceptance of caustic VX hydrolysate. In other words, DuPont Chambers Works is not authorized under its current NPDES permit to treat the Army's caustic VX hydrolysate. DuPont would need to obtain a permit modification from NJDEP to accept this wastestream.

"The incorporation of treatment and disposal of the caustic VX hydrolysate into DuPont's permit would constitute a material and substantive alteration which would require a modification of the existing NPDES permit pursuant to 40 CFR 122.62 (a) (1) since this would be an additional wastestream not addressed in their current permit." NJDEP may initiate the permit modification process (at DuPont's request) by preparing a draft permit incorporating any necessary changes to the existing permit conditions, and making the modified permit available for public comment. In issuing final decision and responding to comment, NJDEP shall give notice of opportunity for public hearing. If DuPont requests a permit modification for the acceptance of the caustic VX hydrolysate at the Chambers Works facility, EPA will work with NJDEP, to ensure that it is protective of human health and the environment.

Finding

- The fact that NJDEP has issued a new NPDES permit for the DuPont SET which specifically prohibits the acceptance of caustic VX hydrolysate until a permit modification is approved, addresses EPA's concern.

Summary of EPA Review

Based on extensive review of the above-mentioned documents and numerous discussions with DuPont, the Army CMA and CDC, EPA believes that all of our previous ecological concerns have been addressed by DuPont and/or the Army. If DuPont requests a modification of its current NJPDES permit for the acceptance of caustic VX hydrolysate, EPA will act in our oversight role to ensure that the treated effluent meets the permit limitations set to protect the environment. Additionally, EPA will make every effort to provide relevant information and participate, as necessary, as DuPont proceeds with its ecological baseline project for the Delaware River.

Section 5. Other Observations

Potential Impact of the DuPont Effluent Discharge on Drinking Water

DuPont performed studies on the effluent stream to the Delaware River from Chambers Works in 1984. At that time, DuPont was discharging 64 million gallons per day and currently the rate is 32 million gallons per day. They performed seven studies in the tidal exchange in the late1980s and a low flow study addendum in 1990. The closest drinking water plant intake, Stanton Water Plant at United Water, is located on the Christina River, greater than 9 miles upstream from the Chambers Works discharge. The low flow condition for the Christina River is 87 million gallons per day. These models showed dilution ratios under low flow (river) conditions. Subsequently, 7-day dye studies were done that confirmed the dilution patterns suggested by the models.

One DuPont study showed spatial relationships of the area water intakes and plant discharge. Plots of the isopleths (equal concentration contours) for the dye concentrations at various locations in the river were presented to CDC. Under normal Delaware River flow conditions, flow from the DuPont waste treatment plant outfall would be downstream from the Stanton potable water intake. To reach this intake with surviving VX would take a combination of events thought to be unlikely. The Newport clearance procedures would have to fail in some manner, and such failure would have to be missed by DuPont in their review of the waste characterization before shipment. Also, these mutual failures would have to occur during a drought condition. As discussed previously, even under these circumstances, and with less than observed pretreatment efficiency at DuPont and no allowance for any other treatment removal or environmental degradation, the concentrations of VX would not pose a significant health risk at the nearest drinking water intake.

Area water basin characteristics were reviewed for this report.

Spatial and flow conditions plus the robustness of the DuPont process are key factors that show that local drinking water supplies will not be adversely impacted.

DuPont Process Management Review

If this proposal is implemented, DuPont, as a regulated treatment, storage and disposal facility (TSDF) in the state of New Jersey, will be required to obtain assurance from NECDF that any material being processed through their facility has been reliably characterized and remains within limits demonstrated during their treatability studies. Before agreeing to treat a client's generated waste, DuPont's Waste Acceptance Laboratory typically analyzes a sample of the waste to characterize certain key parameters and to conduct a laboratory-scale treatability study. If found compatible and acceptable for treatment at DuPont's plant, this initial characterization would serve as a basis for development of a waste characterization profile that the generator would have to conform with for future deliveries to the plant.

The Resource Conservation and Recovery Act of 1976 (RCRA) requires an update on the waste characterization profile at least every 2 years; DuPont routinely performs an update at least once a year. CDC expects that DuPont will update the profile for the CVXH, as it will be 9 to 18 months before they can operate. DuPont does not perform a test or detailed analysis on each batch; therefore, DuPont relies on the waste characterization with the previously mentioned periodic updates. If material is stored for a long period of time (that is, for more than 1 year), DuPont would require it be analytically retested; however, this is not a RCRA issue, but an internal DuPont policy.

The treatability tests were conducted to determine the Chambers Works' range of feed rates to give DuPont an idea of their flexibility in running CVXH material. DuPont performed a statistical analysis on the CVXH from the test results. From that information, they specified five criteria to test and eight key operating parameters. DuPont will generate the final waste characterization and update it as needed to reflect changes in the feedstock from NECDF. The process used by DuPont for the Aberdeen, Maryland, caustic mustard hydrolysate is shown in Figure 2 (provided by DuPont).

DuPont has conducted periodic site visits to NECDF and anticipates quarterly visits after contract award as part of their onsite presence. DuPont has already commented on certain issues, such as the isotainer design and QA/QC reviews. Currently and, after contract award, DuPont will review key documents and changes to ensure they do not affect the waste characterization. As stated previously, it has been recommended that NECDF develop a contingency plan to sample the storage containers if concerns develop or as DuPont needs to update their waste characterization profiles.

Safeguards for Production and Acceptance of Aberdeen Waste

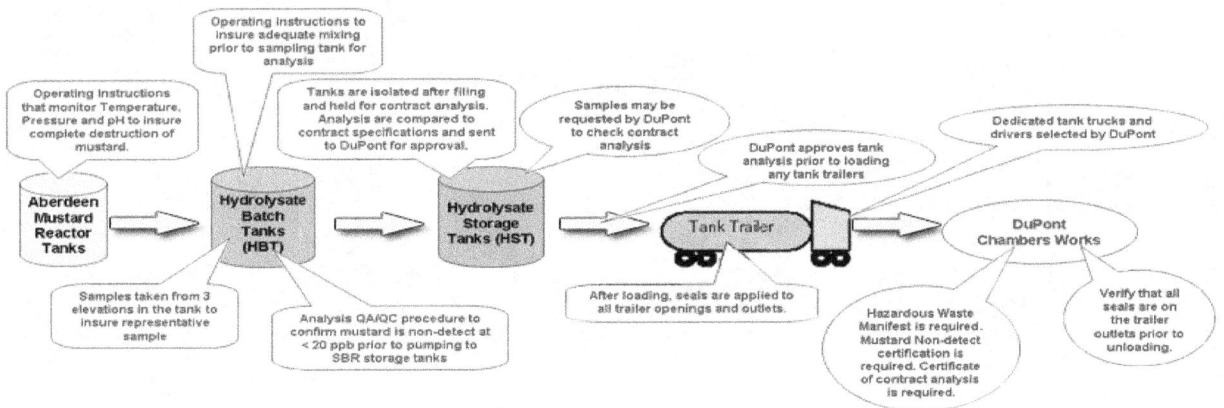

Figure 2 - DuPont Safeguards for Acceptance of Waste Used for Aberdeen Process

This page is intentionally blank

Section 6. Oversight and Safeguard Mechanisms

NECDF Basis of Operation

Since the original review of this proposal, information relevant to the production of CVXH has been developed to support full implementation of processing at NECDF. Following a ramp-up plan approved by the Army, NECDF started processing agent VX on May 5, 2005. The hydrolysate produced is being stored on site at NECDF pending approval of the DuPont proposal.

The NECDF neutralization method is the first non-incineration technology used to process VX in a full-scale facility. Pilot plants, by design, are anticipated to experience the need for frequent process tuning and technical modification as a part of start-up and operation. Examples of technical issues identified to date include a) the need to better match materials of construction used for valves and other components handling VX and CVXH, b) the need to eliminate the potential flammability characteristic from CVXH and still meet clearance criteria, and c) the need to improve sampling to provide a reliable and repeatable representative sample for shipping analysis.

These issues and others have been and will continue to be identified as the plant moves toward full-scale processing. The Army's operations contractor, Parsons, develops strategies to address such issues. CDC and other oversight organizations are charged with the evaluation of Parson's strategies and means for effective resolution of these issues. A number of control and regulatory mechanisms are in place to address any proposed modifications responding to the above issues and future issues. Several of these mechanisms are described as follows.

CDC Chemical Agent Disposal Oversight Background

CDC begins its oversight function for the disposal of a chemical agent by reviewing the Army's proposed destruction technology. CDC focuses on the prevention of agent incidents, advocating a mainline defense consisting of engineering controls (for example, air monitoring, containment, and abatement), then other methods such as emergency response plans, medical provisions, and other procedural and administrative controls. To accomplish the review of the studies, CDC requires documentation sufficiently comprehensive to understand completely the health and safety risks and protections for the facility involved in start-up, operations, and maintenance. This documentation includes the following:

1.   Technological approach and methodology.

2.   Design requirements, standards, and regulations.

3.   Health/risk assessment (including operational risk) criteria, approach/methodology (including basis for methodology and personnel), schedule and public communication.

4.   Design completion schedule.

During operations at chemical weapons destruction facilities, CDC conducts periodic on-site safety reviews. CDC examines facility design provisions and operating procedures that are to protect the workforce and surrounding communities. As part of its oversight role, CDC has often partnered with various state and local agencies, such as state health departments, local medical facilities, and state environmental departments.

During the past 2 years, CDC has reviewed the proposed process and observed selected integrated operations demonstrations to assess the facility and staff's state of readiness for actual agent operations. CDC continues to work closely with the Army and the NECDF team to oversee operational demonstrations, review new team findings, and finalize resolutions.

Regulatory Reviews

Indiana Regulatory Review

After start of agent operations (May 5, 2005), the Indiana Department of Environmental Management (IDEM) has (currently on a weekly basis) conducted RCRA and Hazardous Waste Management compliance inspections of NECDF. In addition, IDEM and NECDF meet routinely to discuss on-going as well as upcoming site-specific activities and possible changes. IDEM does not require any specific approval for operation at full capacity. Instead, IDEM has routinely met with NECDF environmental personnel to stay abreast of any operational or compliance changes and conducted compliance inspections early and routinely (with the frequency based on level of NECDF waste activities). IDEM inspections have included RCRA/Hazardous Waste and other environmental compliance (for example, storm water, air, and erosion control) inspections without distinguishing between full capacity and pilot scale.

NJ Regulatory Review

Any significant changes in the CVXH waste profiles being sent to DuPont or modifications to DuPont's process would need approval from the New Jersey Department of Environmental Protection if it affected the environmental permit.

Process Change Management

CDC focuses on the management systems and looks for "characteristics of a good management system." These characteristics include a) a clear definition of process change and replacement-in-kind, b) a process change risk-ranking or risk-screening system, c) control of changes initiated by the work authorization system, d) control of new chemicals and spare parts through purchasing procedures, and e) consideration of equipment decommissioning. A key area for effective management is how the site deals with process change both from a design and operations standpoint.

Due to the complex nature of the processing issues at the Newport facility, CDC acted as co-lead, along with an Army representative, of a team with members of various expertise (known as a Tiger Team) focusing on medical and worker safety. One area that CDC had been concerned with was change management. CDC stated that "Procedures to allow for process changes need to be well established and documented to allow for proper review and consideration during agent operations." Parsons developed a review program that manages changes to configuration control items, such as the operational procedures, technical design, safety, and environmental documents. These changes require significant review, authorization, and approval by the management review board (MRB). The MRB consists of the management and technical managers and team leads at NECDF. Changes that impact regulatory requirements or facility permits require an even more lengthy review cycle, including the necessary regulatory authority approval.

As part of the oversight role, CDC has had the opportunity to observe the approach that the contractor, Parsons, uses at NECDF. For example, the materials of construction for the reactor valves and gaskets initially resulted in a spill of CVXH in the contained area of the Toxic Cubicle (under engineering controls). This incident eventually required significant modification to the process to replace the valves. These modifications took from June until September 2005 to complete. During this time, the site performed temporary modifications with input from safety, operations, engineering, environmental, and stakeholders to evaluate the path forward.

Concurrently, NECDF found the produced hydrolysate met the criteria for flammability, which required further modification to the equipment and to the process. A detailed plan to design, train workers, install changes, and test the new modifications was developed and reviewed by the MRB and the identified reviewers from safety, maintenance, operations, environmental, training, and medical. Also during this time, changes were made to the review process to ensure lessons learned were incorporated, and proper training for operations and emergency response was identified.

As with the destruction process, the management and change processes continue to evolve. CDC has encouraged NECDF and other chemical weapons disposal sites to follow the recommendations of the U.S. Chemical Safety and Hazard Investigation in a 2001 Safety Bulletin on Management of Change (6). In that bulletin, CSB states the following:

> "The Occupational Safety and Health Administration's (OSHA) Process Safety Management standard and the U.S. Environmental Protection Agency's (EPA) Risk Management Plan require covered facilities to manage changes systematically. It is good practice to do so, irrespective of the specific regulatory requirements."

CDC has stated that procedures to allow for process changes need to be well established and documented to enable proper review and consideration during agent operations. The NECDF team has made significant progress in a) addressing issues that have been raised, b) focusing on safety and health, and c) establishing a balanced team with good working relationships. CDC will continue to monitor their progress as part of its oversight responsibilities.

CONCLUSIONS

In summary, through a focused and combined effort of all parties involved in this review, either as reviewers, or data producers, all the issues identified during the Phase I report have been addressed.

It has been demonstrated that DuPont's modified process was effective, on the laboratory scale, in removing phosphonates and eliminating VX and EA 2192 contaminants if present. During the summer of 2005, DuPont completed testing done to meet EPA's data needs for assessing the potential ecological impact on the Delaware River. EPA believes that all of its previous ecological concerns have been addressed by DuPont and/or the Army. If DuPont requests a modification of its current NJPDES permit for the acceptance of VX hydrolysate, EPA will act in its oversight role to ensure that the treated effluent meets the permit limitations set to protect the environment. Additionally, EPA will make every effort to provide relevant information and to participate, as necessary, while DuPont proceeds with its ecological baseline project for the Delaware River.

CDC and EPA recommend the following:

- NECDF should continue to collect performance data on representative sampling, and provide them to CDC for review, to maintain statistical confidence that representative hydrolysate samples are being collected consistently over time and from varying hydrolysate batches.
- Considering the potential need to re-characterize the CVXH, NECDF needs to develop an effective means to adequately sample the storage containers. CDC believes there is a need to determine what impact, if any, long-term storage will have on the material's characteristics and its conformance to the clearance criteria. In addition, DuPont will likely require new samples and analysis if storage of greater than one year occurs.

- EPA recommends that bioassessment studies be conducted in-stream by DuPont to establish baseline in-stream benthic macroinvertebrate and fish community structure in the vicinity, including downstream of the DuPont discharge, before CVXH processing begins.

DuPont has developed a waste characterization of the NECDF CVXH and identified five characteristics in addition to the flammability and concentration of VX and EA 2192 that are critical to the process. NECDF will need to consistently produce material to meet these criteria and must maintain the quality and consistency of the method of sampling and analysis to ensure the clearance criteria can be reliably verified and characterized to the satisfaction of DuPont and the regulatory states involved. Additionally, considering the potentially long storage time for the CVXH, NECDF needs to develop contingency plans to adequately sample the storage containers if the need arises. The impact, if any, such storage will have on the identified criteria and the material's characteristics is not yet understood and an effective means to provide samples to ensure the material has not changed significantly is necessary.

If this proposal is accepted by the regulatory officials, regulatory and procedural mechanisms will need to be finalized to ensure that all clearance and acceptance criteria specified by DuPont and the state of New Jersey are met throughout the life of the project. Adequate oversight and safeguard mechanisms, especially in the area of change management, sampling, and communication between DuPont and NECDF will need further development and refinement to ensure ongoing protection for public health, safety, and the environment throughout the life of the project.

REFERENCES

1. Centers for Disease Control and Prevention. Review of the U.S. Army proposal for off-site treatment and disposal of caustic VX hydrolysate from the Newport Chemical Agent Disposal Facility. Atlanta (GA): US Department of Health and Human Services; Apr 2005.

2. Lawler, Matusky and Skelly Engineers. Task A. II report preliminary assessment of Nearfield dilution of Chambers Works discharge in the Delaware River. Pearl River (NY): 1989–1990: 10965. Prepared for E.I. DuPont & Company.

3. Science Applications International Corporation. Effect of the DuPont persulfate treatment process on trace quantities of VX and EA 2192 in hydrolysate. Edgewood, Maryland: Science Applications International Corporation; Aug 2005.

4. Carmagen Engineering, Inc. Assessment of the treatability of caustic VX hydrolysate at the DuPont Secure Environmental Treatment Facility. Atlanta: US Department of Health and Human Services, Centers for Disease Control and Prevention; Jan 2006.

5. E.I. DuPont & Company. Treatability study summary for phosphonate removal technology on 16% Newport (IN) caustic hydrolysate. Wilmington, Delaware: E.I. DuPont & Company; Aug 2005.

6. US Chemical Hazards and Safety Investigation Board. Management of change. Washington (DC): US Chemical Hazards and Safety Investigation Board; Aug 2001. (Safety bulletin no. 201-04-SB). Available at: http://www.csb.gov/safety_publications/docs/moc082801.pdf.

Attachment 1

List of Abbreviations

Carmagen	Carmagen Engineering, Inc.
CDC	Centers for Disease Control and Prevention
CVXH	Caustic VX hydrolysate (equivalent to VX hydrolysate or Newport caustic hydrolysate)
DCC	dicyclohexyldicarbodiimide
DIC	diisopropylcarbodiimide
EA 2192	S-[2-diisopropylaminoethyl] methylphosphonothioic acid
EAS	Environmental Assessment Statement
EMPA	ethyl methylphosphonic acid
EPA	U.S. Environmental Protection Agency
°F	degrees Fahrenheit
FONSI	Finding of No Significant Impact
gpd	gallons per day
IDEM	Indiana Department of Environmental Management
LOQ	limit of quantification
MDL	method detection limit [EPA defined]
MPA	methylphosphonic acid
MRB	management review board
NCEH	National Center for Environmental Health
NCH	Newport (Indiana) caustic hydrolysate (equivalent to caustic VX hydrolysate)
NECDF	Newport Chemical Agent Disposal Facility
NJDEP	New Jersey Department of Environmental Protection
NJPDES	New Jersey Pollution Discharge Elimination System
NPDES	National Pollutant Discharge Elimination System
ORD	Office of Research and Development
OSHA	Occupational Safety and Health Administration
PACT®	Powdered Activated Carbon Treatment System
ppb	parts per billion
ppm	parts per million
QA/QC	quality assurance/quality control
QC	quality control
RCRA	Resource Conservation and Recovery Act of 1976 (amended 1984)
SET	[DuPont] Secure Environmental Treatment [Chamber Works]

SLERA	Screening Level Ecological Risk Assessment
EPA	U.S. Environmental Protection Agency
VX	O-ethyl S-([2-(diisopropylamino) ethyl)] methyl phosphonothioate
WET	Whole effluent toxicity